The Hidden Current of Health

Navigating May-Thurner Syndrome
and the Rivers of Vascular Wellness

Dennis J. Bell

Copyright

This page belongs to

Table of Contents

Introduction

Welcome to "Unveiling May-Thurner Syndrome: A Comprehensive Guide to Understanding and Managing Vascular Health." In the following pages, I will unravel the mysteries of May-Thurner Syndrome (MTS) and examine the complexities of vascular health. Whether you are a medical practitioner, a patient seeking knowledge, or simply inquisitive about the complexities of the human body, this ebook will provide you with useful insights and actionable information.

The vascular system, which includes arteries, veins, and capillaries, is the human body's lifeline, transporting oxygen and nutrition to tissues and organs while eliminating waste materials. This intricate network is critical to sustaining general health and well-being, impacting a variety of biological activities such as circulation and blood pressure management, immunological response, and tissue repair.

Given the vascular system's crucial importance, it is understandable that any interruption or dysfunction can have serious implications. Vascular diseases include a wide range of conditions, from minor problems like varicose veins to more serious conditions like peripheral artery disease and deep vein thrombosis.

Among the various vascular disorders, May-Thurner Syndrome stands out as a relatively unknown yet significant entity. MTS, also known as iliac vein compression syndrome or Cockett syndrome, is defined by the compression of the left common iliac vein against the lumbar spine caused by the overlaying right common iliac artery. This anatomical aberration can cause a variety of symptoms and problems, such as deep vein thrombosis (DVT), chronic venous insufficiency, and pulmonary embolism.

Despite its clinical relevance, May-Thurner Syndrome frequently goes undetected or misdiagnosed. The subtle nature of its symptoms, which can be mistaken for those of other vascular illnesses, combined with a lack of awareness among healthcare professionals and the general public, contribute to its underdiagnosis and treatment.

Given the aforementioned difficulties and the increasing significance of vascular health, the goal of this ebook is to provide you with information and insight on May-Thurner Syndrome. This resource is intended to meet the needs of individuals who are interested in protecting their vascular health, patients who are having trouble explaining their symptoms, or healthcare providers who want to improve their diagnostic skills.

To demystify May-Thurner Syndrome, I will first provide a thorough description of its genesis, clinical presentation, and therapy techniques. Secondly, I hope to promote a more general awareness of vascular health and its implications for overall wellness. Through an examination of the complexities surrounding MTS and a wider examination of vascular physiology and pathology, our goal is to provide you with the knowledge and understanding needed to successfully negotiate the challenging field of vascular medicine.

I will go on an exploration and discovery journey throughout the upcoming chapters, supported by clinical knowledge and evidence-based ideas. To prepare for a more thorough examination of May-Thurner Syndrome, I will begin by providing an outline of the vascular system and typical vascular disorders.

Every chapter provides insightful information and useful advice, covering everything from comprehending the fundamental origins and risk factors of MTS to clarifying its clinical presentations and possible complications. To enable you to take proactive measures toward ideal vascular health, I will examine diagnostic techniques, therapeutic modalities, and preventive tactics.

Furthermore, I will look at lifestyle variables and behavioral choices that might impact vascular health, emphasizing the need for holistic approaches to health maintenance and illness prevention. By raising awareness and education, I hope to empower people to be proactive stewards of their vascular health, advocating for themselves and their loved ones in the quest for well-being.

As I begin this journey together, I encourage you to explore the pages ahead with curiosity, openness, and a passion for knowledge. Whether you are a seasoned healthcare professional, a freshly diagnosed patient, or simply a curious mind eager to discover the wonders of the human body, there is something for everyone.

So, let us go on this journey of discovery, armed with inquiry tools, an exploratory spirit, and a desire to comprehend. I will unravel the mysteries of May-Thurner Syndrome and light the road to good vascular health. Welcome aboard!

Chapter 1

Understanding Vascular Health

In this chapter, I will study the complex world of vascular health. I will look at the anatomy and physiology of the vascular system, unraveling its intricacies and revealing its critical role in preserving general health. From the small capillaries to the massive arteries and veins, I will look at the inner workings of this critical network and its far-reaching ramifications for human health.

Overview of the Vascular System

The vascular system also called the circulatory system, is a huge network of blood vessels that convey blood throughout the body. It comprises three types of vessels: arteries, veins, and capillaries. Arteries transport oxygenated blood out from the heart to various tissues and organs, whereas veins return oxygen-depleted blood to the heart. Capillaries, the tiniest and most numerous vessels, aid in the exchange of nutrients and wastes between blood and tissues.

Arteries: The Pathways of Oxygen

Arteries are responsible for transporting oxygenated blood from the heart to the body's tissues and organs.

They have strong, elastic walls made of smooth muscle and connective tissue, which allows them to resist the enormous pressure produced by the heart's pumping motion. Arteries branch into smaller vessels called arterioles, which deliver blood to specific parts of the body.

Veins: The Return Path to the Heart

Veins bring deoxygenated blood back to the heart for reoxygenation. Veins, unlike arteries, have thinner walls and less elastic tissue because they work at lower pressures. Veins have one-way valves that prohibit backward flow and ensure unidirectional blood flow, allowing blood to return to the heart more quickly. This mechanism is especially significant in the context of chronic venous insufficiency, in which valve malfunction causes venous congestion and edema.

Capillaries: The Site of Exchange

Capillaries serve as the contact between the circulatory system and the body's tissues. These small capillaries form intricate networks within organs and tissues, allowing for the movement of gasses, nutrients, and waste products between blood and cells. Capillary walls consist of a single layer of endothelial cells, allowing chemicals to diffuse efficiently across the vessel wall. This intricate network of capillaries guarantees that all cells in the body receive the nutrition and oxygen they require while also removing metabolic waste.

Common Vascular Conditions

Despite its remarkable resilience and adaptability, the vascular system is susceptible to a wide range of disorders and diseases. These disorders can affect any portion of the circulatory system, including the smallest capillary and the largest artery or vein. Understanding these common vascular disorders is critical for recognizing symptoms, effectively diagnosing them, and implementing effective treatment plans.

Atherosclerosis: The Silent Threat

Atherosclerosis is a progressive disorder marked by the accumulation of plaque within the walls of arteries. This plaque is made up of cholesterol, fatty acids, calcium, and other components that slowly collect and constrict the artery lumen, limiting blood flow. Over time, atherosclerosis can cause arterial blockages or plaques, raising the risk of heart attack, stroke, and peripheral artery disease.

Deep Vein Thrombosis (DVT): A Clot in the Shadows

Deep vein thrombosis (DVT) happens when a blood clot forms within the body's deep veins, usually in the legs or pelvis. This syndrome can result from a variety of circumstances, including prolonged immobilization, surgery, trauma, or underlying medical issues. If left untreated, DVT can lead to major complications such as pulmonary embolism (PE), which occurs when a clot breaks free and travels to the lungs, producing potentially fatal complications.

Varicose Veins: Aesthetic Nuisance or Medical Concern?

Varicose veins are big, twisted veins that appear blue or purple beneath the skin's surface. They mostly affect the legs and feet and are frequently accompanied by symptoms such as pain, swelling, and discomfort. While varicose veins are commonly regarded as a cosmetic issue, they can also suggest underlying venous insufficiency or dysfunction, necessitating medical intervention to avoid complications.

Peripheral Artery Disease (PAD): The Impaired Pathway

Peripheral artery disease (PAD) is a vascular illness defined by the narrowing or blocking of arteries in the extremities, most commonly the legs. This reduction in blood flow can cause leg pain, cramping, and weakness, especially during strenuous exertion. Left untreated, PAD can lead to more serious problems such as tissue damage, non-healing wounds, and limb ischemia.

Understanding May-Thurner Syndrome

May-Thurner Syndrome (MTS) is a lesser-known but clinically relevant illness that falls under the category of vascular disorders. In the next chapters, I will delve into the complexities of MTS, including its origin, clinical symptoms, diagnostic strategies, and therapeutic choices. I will reveal the complexities of this ailment and equip you to recognize its indications and symptoms through extensive explanations supported by medical research and case studies.

What Sets MTS Apart?

May-Thurner Syndrome is defined by the compression of the left common iliac vein by the overlaying right common iliac artery, which causes venous outflow blockage and other symptoms. Unlike other vascular disorders, MTS frequently presents with nonspecific symptoms, making it difficult to identify without a high level of suspicion. Understanding the distinct anatomical and physiological characteristics of MTS allows healthcare providers to better recognize and manage the illness in clinical practice.

The Impact of MTS on Vascular Health

MTS can have far-reaching effects on vascular health, predisposing people to issues like deep vein thrombosis (DVT) and chronic venous insufficiency (CVI). MTS, which blocks venous blood flow and impairs normal circulation, can contribute to the development of severe symptoms and lower patients' quality of life. Recognizing the potential effects of MTS is critical for carrying out prompt interventions and avoiding long-term difficulties.

Diagnostic Challenges and Strategies

MTS is difficult to diagnose because of its nonspecific symptoms and clinical presentations that overlap with other vascular diseases. However, numerous diagnostic modalities, including imaging procedures like venography and intravascular ultrasonography (IVUS), can help confirm the diagnosis of MTS. Healthcare practitioners can enhance diagnostic accuracy and patient outcomes by using a systematic evaluation strategy that incorporates clinical judgment.

Treatment Approaches and Considerations

May-Thurner Syndrome is normally managed using a multidisciplinary approach to ease venous blockage, treat symptoms, and prevent consequences. Conservative methods, such as compression therapy and lifestyle changes, may be suggested as initial interventions. However, in cases of significant venous obstruction or recurring symptoms, more intrusive therapies, such as endovascular stenting or surgical venous reconstruction, may be required to restore normal venous flow and enhance patient outcomes.

This chapter established the groundwork for our research on vascular health and May-Thurner Syndrome. Understanding the anatomy and physiology of the vascular system, as well as becoming familiar with typical vascular diseases, prepares us to recognize the complexity of MTS and its consequences for patient management.

Chapter 2

Causes and Risk Factors of May-Thurner Syndrome

This chapter explores the fundamental causes of May-Thurner Syndrome (MTS) and its risk factors. By understanding the anatomical predispositions, genetic influences, and environmental factors that contribute to the development of MTS, I can better identify at-risk individuals and implement preventive measures to mitigate their risk. Through a comprehensive exploration of the etiology and pathogenesis of MTS, supported by medical research and clinical evidence, I aim to shed light on this often overlooked vascular condition.

Anatomical Factors: Understanding the Anatomy of MTS

May-Thurner Syndrome is defined by the compression of the left common iliac vein (LCIV) between the right common iliac artery (RCIA) and the lumbar spine. This anatomical anomaly occurs when these structures are close together in the pelvis, causing mechanical compression of the LCIV during moments of elevated intra-abdominal pressure, such as respiration or physical activity.

The Cockett's Compression Point: A Vulnerable Junction

The point of compression, also known as Cockett's compression point, is usually seen around the pelvic brim, where the RCIA passes over the LCIV. This anatomical shape predisposes the LCIV to extrinsic compression by pulsatile arterial flow, which worsens venous stasis and promotes the production of thrombi inside the vascular lumen.

Variations in Anatomy: The Role of Anatomical Variants

While compression of the LCIV by the RCIA is thought to be characteristic of MTS, differences in pelvic anatomy can affect the syndrome's severity and presentation. Anatomical variations such as an abnormal course of the iliac arteries, asymmetrical pelvic architecture, or congenital malformations might worsen venous compression and predispose people to symptomatic MTS.

Risk Factors for May-Thurner Syndrome

In addition to anatomical predispositions, various risk factors have been identified as increasing the probability of developing May-Thurner Syndrome. These risk factors include genetic, physiological, and environmental variables that cause venous stasis, endothelial damage, and hypercoagulability, predisposing people to venous thrombosis and venous outflow blockage.

Gender Disparities: The Female Predilection

Studies consistently reveal that girls have a higher prevalence of MTS than males, with a female-to-male ratio ranging from 2:1 to 5:1. This gender gap is assumed to be due to hormonal factors, specifically estrogen, which has been linked to venous dilation, endothelial dysfunction, and hypercoagulability.

Pregnancy and Hormonal Factors: Unravelling the Hormonal Link

Pregnancy is a substantial risk factor for the development of MTS, as hormonal changes during pregnancy contribute to venous congestion and compression. Elevated levels of estrogen and progesterone during pregnancy cause venous dilatation and wall relaxation, predisposing women to venous stasis and thrombosis.

Congenital Anomalies: Inherited Predispositions

Genetic factors play an important part in the etiology of MTS, with familial clustering and hereditary predispositions seen in some cases. Mutations or changes in genes linked to venous formation, hemostasis, and vascular integrity may predispose people to venous abnormalities, putting them at risk for MTS and other venous illnesses.

Chronic Conditions: The Impact of Chronic Illness

Chronic medical problems such as obesity, hypertension, diabetes, and autoimmune illnesses have been linked to an increased risk of MTS. These disorders can increase the risk of endothelial dysfunction, inflammation, and metabolic abnormalities, all of which contribute to venous thrombosis and insufficiency.

Lifestyle Factors: The Influence of Sedentary Behavior

Sedentary lifestyle behaviors, such as extended sitting or immobility, have been associated with venous stasis and thrombosis, which raises the risk of MTS. Individuals who spend lengthy periods seated, such as office workers, long-distance travelers, or those with mobility impairments, are more susceptible to venous compression and decreased venous return.

Clinical Implications and Diagnostic Considerations

Understanding the origins and risk factors of May-Thurner Syndrome is critical for identifying at-risk patients and adopting effective diagnostic procedures. By identifying anatomical predispositions, genetic influences, and environmental factors that contribute to the development of MTS, healthcare providers can tailor their approach to patient evaluation and management, improving patient outcomes and lowering the burden of this frequently overlooked vascular condition.

Recognizing the Red Flags: Clinical Presentations of MTS

May-Thurner Syndrome can cause a variety of symptoms, including unilateral limb pain, edema, heaviness, and weariness. These symptoms are frequently exacerbated by extended standing or physical activity and can worsen over time if not managed. Recognizing the distinctive clinical symptoms of MTS is critical for distinguishing it from other vascular diseases and directing appropriate diagnostic examination.

Diagnostic Modalities: From Imaging to Intervention

Diagnosing May-Thurner Syndrome often involves a mix of clinical evaluation, imaging studies, and diagnostic tests. Imaging methods such as duplex ultrasonography, computed tomography (CT) angiography, magnetic resonance venography (MRV), and venography can provide precise anatomical information as well as detect venous compression or obstruction. Additionally, intravascular ultrasound (IVUS) and venography may be used to confirm the diagnosis and guide therapeutic interventions, such as venous stenting or angioplasty.

Differential Diagnosis: Distinguishing MTS from Mimics

There are similarities in the clinical symptoms of May-Thurner Syndrome and other vascular disorders such as chronic venous insufficiency (CVI), deep vein thrombosis (DVT), and iliac vein compression caused by other structures. Using a thorough clinical assessment, imaging scans, and laboratory testing, differential diagnosis entails ruling out other etiologies. Healthcare providers can accurately diagnose MTS and commence suitable treatment methods by taking into account the patient's history, symptoms, and diagnostic findings.

In this chapter, I looked at the underlying causes and risk factors for May-Thurner Syndrome, including anatomical predispositions, genetic influences, and environmental factors that contribute to its pathogenesis.

Understanding the complexity of MTS and its clinical implications enables healthcare practitioners to better identify at-risk individuals, apply appropriate diagnostic procedures, and improve patient outcomes. In the following chapters, I will go over the diagnosis, therapy, and management of MTS, giving you full insights and evidence-based suggestions for navigating this complex vascular disorder.

Chapter 3

Symptoms and Complications of May-Thurner Syndrome

In this chapter, I look at the clinical symptoms and probable complications of May-Thurner Syndrome (MTS). Healthcare providers can better diagnose and manage this sometimes ignored vascular disorder by recognizing the range of symptoms associated with MTS, as well as the potential consequences of untreated disease. I hope to provide you with the knowledge and resources they need to enhance patient care and results by thoroughly exploring MTS symptoms, diagnostic considerations, and management techniques, all supported by medical research and clinical data.

Symptoms of May-Thurner Syndrome

May-Thurner Syndrome can cause a wide range of symptoms, which vary in severity and duration. MTS has a generic clinical presentation, with symptoms that overlap with those of other venous illnesses such as deep vein thrombosis (DVT), chronic venous insufficiency (CVI), and peripheral arterial disease (PAD). Recognizing the distinctive symptoms of MTS is critical for guiding diagnostic diagnosis and establishing suitable treatment plans.

Leg Pain and Swelling: A Common Complaint

One of the most common symptoms of May-Thurner Syndrome is unilateral leg discomfort and edema, which usually affects the left lower extremity. This pain might be described as dull, achy, or throbbing, and it may worsen with prolonged standing or physical exercise. Swelling, also known as edema, can accompany leg pain and is usually limited to the affected limb due to venous congestion and poor venous return.

Venous Claudication: The Limb Fatigue

Another typical symptom of May-Thurner Syndrome is venous claudication, often known as limb tiredness. This feeling of heaviness, cramping, or weariness in the affected limb usually develops after physical exertion and is eased by rest. Venous claudication is characterized by poor venous return and can be aggravated by conditions that raise intra-abdominal pressure, such as standing or effort.

Varicose Veins: Visible Signs of Venous Insufficiency
Varicose veins are swollen, twisted veins that commonly appear in the affected limb as a result of venous

congestion and valve malfunction. These superficial veins might appear blue or purple beneath the skin's surface and be accompanied by symptoms like itching, burning, and throbbing. Varicose veins are a visible sign of venous insufficiency and may signal underlying May-Thurner Syndrome or other venous illnesses.

Skin Changes and Ulceration: Signs of Chronic Venous Insufficiency

Chronic venous insufficiency (CVI) can cause progressive changes in the skin on the affected limb, such as discoloration, thickness, and ulceration. Skin alterations might range from minor pigmentation and eczema to more serious problems including venous stasis ulcers. These ulcers usually appear over bony prominences or sites of venous congestion and might take a long time to heal if not treated properly.

Complications of May-Thurner Syndrome

Untreated May-Thurner Syndrome can cause a range of consequences, including acute thrombotic episodes, chronic venous insufficiency, and venous ulcers. Understanding the potential repercussions of MTS is critical for making informed treatment decisions and avoiding long-term morbidity and mortality.

Deep Vein Thrombosis (DVT): A Silent Threat

Deep vein thrombosis (DVT) is a common complication of May-Thurner Syndrome, which is defined as the production of blood clots in the affected limb's deep veins. These clots can disrupt venous flow, causing discomfort, edema, and inflammation. If left untreated, DVT can lead to more serious consequences such as pulmonary embolism (PE), which occurs when a clot dislodges and moves to the lungs, causing potentially fatal breathing compromise.

Pulmonary Embolism (PE): The Consequence of Thromboembolism

Pulmonary embolism (PE) is a significant consequence of May-Thurner Syndrome that occurs when a blood clot from the deep veins enters the lungs and obstructs pulmonary blood flow. PE can cause symptoms such as chest pain, shortness of breath, and hemoptysis, necessitating quick medical attention to avoid morbidity and fatality. Recognizing the signs and symptoms of PE is critical for prompt diagnostic diagnosis and treatment.

Chronic Venous Insufficiency (CVI): The Sequelae of Venous Hypertension

Chronic venous insufficiency (CVI) is a common complication of May-Thurner Syndrome, caused by persistent venous hypertension and decreased venous return. CVI symptoms include leg swelling, discomfort, and skin changes such as pigmentation, eczema, and ulceration. These signs are due to the persistent inflammatory alterations and microvascular dysfunction that accompany venous congestion and stasis.

Venous Ulcers: The Wounds That Won't Heal

Venous ulcers are a serious consequence of May-Thurner Syndrome that results from persistent venous insufficiency and tissue ischemia. These non-healing lesions usually appear on bony prominences or sites of venous congestion and can take a long time to cure if not treated properly. Venous ulcers can have a substantial influence on patients' quality of life, necessitating ongoing wound care and management to promote healing and prevent recurrence.

Diagnostic Evaluation and Management Considerations

May-Thurner Syndrome is diagnosed with a comprehensive patient evaluation that includes a detailed clinical history, physical examination, and diagnostic imaging studies. Recognizing the typical symptoms and potential consequences of MTS allows healthcare providers to conduct appropriate diagnostic evaluations and execute prompt interventions to improve patient outcomes.

Imaging Modalities: From Duplex Ultrasound to Venography

Imaging investigations such as duplex ultrasonography, computed tomography (CT) angiography, magnetic resonance venography (MRV), and venography are critical in identifying May-Thurner Syndrome and evaluating venous anatomy and function. These techniques can provide extensive anatomical information and detect venous compression or obstruction, directing treatment decisions and treatments.

Therapeutic Interventions: From Conservative Measures to Invasive Procedures

May-Thurner Syndrome is normally managed using a multidisciplinary approach to ease venous blockage, treat symptoms, and prevent consequences. Conservative therapies such as compression therapy, elevation, and lifestyle changes may be recommended as initial interventions. However, in cases of significant venous obstruction or recurring symptoms, more intrusive therapies like endovascular stenting or surgical venous reconstruction may be required to restore normal venous flow and enhance patient outcomes.

In this chapter, I looked at the range of symptoms and potential problems associated with May-Thurner Syndrome, emphasizing the necessity of early detection and treatment. Understanding the clinical signs of MTS, as well as the consequences of untreated disease, allows healthcare providers to effectively manage patients with this often ignored vascular ailment and improve outcomes. In the following chapters, I will go over the diagnosis, therapy, and management of MTS, giving you full insights and evidence-based suggestions for navigating this complex vascular disorder.

Chapter 4

Lifestyle Strategies for Vascular Health

This chapter investigates the crucial role of lifestyle variables in supporting vascular health and preventing vascular disease. Lifestyle choices, ranging from regular exercise and healthy eating habits to stress management and tobacco cessation, are critical in maintaining optimal cardiovascular function and lowering the risk of disorders like May-Thurner Syndrome (MTS). Individuals who embrace a holistic approach to health maintenance and illness prevention can empower themselves to take control of their vascular health and live better, more rewarding lives.

Exercise and Physical Activity: The Foundation of Vascular Wellness

Regular exercise and physical activity are essential for vascular health, as they promote cardiovascular fitness, improve circulation, and lower the risk of vascular illnesses. Aerobic exercises like walking, cycling, swimming, and jogging help strengthen the heart and blood arteries, improve blood flow, and lower blood pressure. Incorporating resistance training and flexibility exercises can also boost muscle strength, joint mobility, and functional capacity.

Benefits of Exercise for Vascular Health

Exercise provides numerous benefits for vascular health, including:

- Improved endothelial function: Exercise promotes the synthesis of nitric oxide, a powerful vasodilator that relaxes blood vessels and increases blood flow.
- Reduced inflammation: Regular physical exercise has been shown to reduce systemic inflammation and oxidative stress, both of which are linked to the development of vascular disorders.
- Lower blood pressure: Exercise reduces blood pressure via increasing arterial compliance, decreasing peripheral resistance, and increasing baroreceptor sensitivity.
- Improved lipid profile: Aerobic exercise increases high-density lipoprotein (HDL) cholesterol levels while decreasing low-density lipoprotein (LDL) cholesterol levels, hence improving lipid metabolism and lowering the risk of atherosclerosis.

Recommendations for Exercise Prescription

The American Heart Association recommends at least 150 minutes of moderate-intensity aerobic activity or 75 minutes of vigorous-intensity aerobic exercise per week, as well as two or more days of muscle-strengthening activities. Individuals with pre-existing vascular problems or risk factors should contact their doctor before beginning a new fitness program, and their exercise regimen should be tailored to their unique needs and abilities.

Healthy Diet: Nourishing Your Vascular System

A well-balanced and healthy diet is vital for maintaining vascular health and preventing vascular disorders. Individuals can give their bodies the critical nutrients they require for optimal cardiovascular function and overall well-being by focusing on whole foods, fruits and vegetables, lean proteins, and healthy fats. Key dietary components that enhance vascular health are:

Omega-3 Fatty Acids: The Heart-Healthy Fats

Omega-3 fatty acids, which are present in fatty fish like salmon, mackerel, and sardines, as well as flaxseeds, chia seeds, and walnuts, have been demonstrated to reduce inflammation, lower triglyceride levels, and improve endothelial function. Incorporating omega-3-rich foods into your diet can improve vascular health and lower your risk of atherosclerosis and heart disease.

Antioxidants: Nature's Defense Against Free Radicals

Antioxidant-rich meals include berries, citrus fruits, leafy greens, and colorful vegetables, which are high in vitamins, minerals, and phytonutrients that assist in neutralizing free radicals and minimize oxidative stress. By including antioxidant-rich foods in your diet, you can protect your blood vessels from damage, increase circulation, and promote overall vascular health.

Fiber: The Digestive Dynamo

Dietary fiber helps to maintain healthy cholesterol levels, promotes satiety, and regulates blood sugar levels. Whole grains, legumes, fruits, and vegetables are high in fiber, which can help lower LDL cholesterol, reduce the risk of atherosclerosis, and improve gastrointestinal health. To maximize the advantages of this crucial nutrient, include a range of fiber-rich foods in your diet.

Stress Management: Calming the Waters of Vascular Health

Chronic stress and psychological variables can have a significant impact on vascular health, accelerating the development and progression of vascular disorders. Individuals can lower their risk of vascular disorders like hypertension, atherosclerosis, and MTS by practicing stress management techniques and using good coping skills.

**Key stress management practices include:
Mindfulness Meditation: Cultivating Present-Moment Awareness**

Mindfulness meditation is the practice of focusing your attention on the present moment without judgment, allowing you to examine your thoughts, emotions, and sensations with clarity and equanimity. Mindfulness meditation can help people reduce stress, improve emotional control, and increase resilience to life's obstacles.

Deep Breathing Exercises: Harnessing the Power of Breath

Deep breathing exercises, such as diaphragmatic breathing or belly breathing, can assist activate the body's relaxation response, which lowers heart rate, blood pressure, and muscle tension. Individuals who do deep breathing exercises daily can achieve a state of calm and relaxation, which promotes vascular health and overall well-being.

Physical Activity: Energizing the Mind and Body

Regular physical activity is not only good for your arteries, but it also helps you handle stress and feel better emotionally. Aerobic exercises like walking, jogging, and cycling can help produce endorphins, neurotransmitters that increase feelings of enjoyment and relaxation, while also lowering cortisol levels, the body's major stress hormone.

Tobacco Cessation: Breaking Free from the Grip of Addiction

Tobacco smoking is a substantial risk factor for vascular illnesses such as atherosclerosis, peripheral artery disease (PAD), and May-Thurner syndrome. Quitting smoking or using tobacco products can considerably lower the chance of developing vascular diseases while also improving general health and well-being. Quitting smoking is one of the most essential steps people can take to improve their cardiovascular health and extend their lives.

Benefits of Tobacco Cessation for Vascular Health

Quitting smoking has many advantages for vascular health, including:

- Reduced risk of atherosclerosis: Smoking harms the endothelium lining of blood vessels, increases inflammation, and hastens the course of atherosclerosis. Quitting smoking reduces the chance of acquiring arterial plaque and coronary artery disease.

- Improved circulation: Smoking constricts blood vessels and decreases blood flow, raising the risk of peripheral arterial disease (PAD) and venous insufficiency. Quitting smoking improves circulation, increases tissue oxygenation, and lowers the incidence of vascular problems.

- Reduced blood pressure: Smoking raises blood pressure and heart rate, putting more strain on the cardiovascular system and raising the risk of hypertension and stroke. Quitting smoking can lower blood pressure and lessen the risk of cardiovascular events.

In this chapter, I looked at the importance of lifestyle variables in improving vascular health and preventing vascular disorders. Individuals can empower themselves to take charge of their vascular health by adopting healthy behaviors such as regular exercise, a balanced diet, stress management strategies, and smoke cessation. In the following chapters, I will go over the diagnosis, therapy, and management of MTS, giving you full insights and evidence-based suggestions for navigating this complex vascular disorder.

Chapter 5

Lifestyle Strategies for Vascular Health

I move our attention to the significance of behavioral decisions and lifestyle factors in maintaining vascular health and preventing vascular disorders in this crucial chapter. I will look at evidence-based measures for improving vascular function and lowering the risk of cardiovascular problems, including the value of regular exercise and physical activity, as well as the impact of dietary choices and stress management techniques. Drawing on the most recent research findings and clinical advice, I hope to provide you with practical insights and actionable actions toward a heart-healthy lifestyle.

Exercise and Physical Activity

Regular exercise is widely acknowledged as one of the most important components of cardiovascular health, with benefits for vascular function, blood pressure regulation, and overall cardiovascular fitness. Aerobic exercises like walking, running, cycling, and swimming have been found to improve endothelial function, increase blood flow, and lower arterial stiffness. Resistance training and weight-bearing activities can also help you retain muscle mass, enhance insulin sensitivity, and support metabolic health.

Guidelines for Physical Activity

The American Heart Association recommends at least 150 minutes of moderate-intensity aerobic activity or 75 minutes of vigorous-intensity aerobic exercise per week, with muscle-strengthening activities added on two or more days. These guidelines emphasize the need to mix a range of activities into one's regimen, including aerobic and weight training exercises, to obtain overall cardiovascular benefits.

Benefits of Exercise on Vascular Health

Regular physical activity has been demonstrated to have a variety of benefits for vascular health, including improved endothelial function, increased vasodilation, and decreased arterial stiffness. Exercise-induced vascular adaptations, such as increased nitric oxide production and endothelial repair mechanisms, help to improve blood flow, reduce inflammation, and lower blood pressure. Furthermore, regular exercise can help reduce risk factors for cardiovascular disease such as obesity, diabetes, and dyslipidemia, lowering the likelihood of developing vascular problems.

Healthy Diet

Dietary habits have a significant impact on vascular health by altering parameters such as blood pressure, cholesterol levels, and inflammation. A heart-healthy diet rich in fruits and vegetables, whole grains, lean meats, and healthy fats can help keep arteries healthy and lower the risk of atherosclerosis and other vascular illnesses. Key components of a vascular-friendly diet are:

Mediterranean Diet

The Mediterranean diet, which includes plenty of fruits and vegetables, whole grains, olive oil, nuts, seeds, and fish, has been linked to a variety of cardiovascular advantages. The Mediterranean diet is high in antioxidants, anti-inflammatory chemicals, and omega-3 fatty acids, which enhance vascular health by lowering oxidative stress, inflammation, and LDL cholesterol levels. Furthermore, this dietary pattern prioritizes plant-based meals while minimizing processed foods, sugar, and saturated fats, which promotes cardiovascular health.

DASH Diet

The Dietary Approaches to Stop Hypertension (DASH) diet is intended to lower blood pressure and reduce the risk of hypertension-related problems. It promotes eating fruits and vegetables, whole grains, lean proteins, and low-fat dairy products while limiting sodium intake and avoiding processed meals, red meat, and sugary beverages. The DASH diet promotes a nutrient-dense, low-sodium diet, which helps maintain vascular tone, minimize arterial stiffness, and enhance overall cardiovascular function.

Stress Management Techniques

Chronic stress can harm vascular health, increasing hypertension, inflammation, and endothelial dysfunction. Stress management practices such as mindfulness meditation, deep breathing exercises, yoga, and progressive muscle relaxation can assist in reducing the physiological and psychological impacts of stress and boosting vascular well-being. These activities promote relaxation, mental clarity, and resilience in the face of life's obstacles, resulting in a sense of balance and well-being.

Mindfulness Meditation

Mindfulness meditation entails practicing present-moment mindfulness and nonjudgmental acceptance of one's thoughts, emotions, and bodily sensations. Individuals who practice mindfulness meditation regularly can increase their emotional resilience, lower their response to stimuli, and create an inner sense of peace and equanimity. Furthermore, mindfulness-based stress reduction programs have been demonstrated to lower blood pressure, lower inflammation markers, and increase endothelial function, indicating that this practice may have vascular health advantages.

Deep Breathing Exercises

Deep breathing exercises, such as diaphragmatic and paced breathing, use slow, rhythmic inhalation and exhalation techniques to activate the parasympathetic nervous system and induce relaxation. Deep breathing techniques, which slow the respiratory rate and extend the exhalation phase, can create feelings of relaxation, reduce sympathetic nervous system activity, and drop heart rate and blood pressure. These approaches are simple to implement into everyday routines and are effective tools for stress management and vascular health promotion.

As I close this Chapter, I have emphasized the importance of lifestyle variables in shaping vascular health and preventing cardiovascular disease. From the cardiovascular advantages of regular exercise and physical activity to the effects of dietary choices and stress management approaches, I have identified evidence-based ways to improve vascular function and lower the risk of vascular problems. I hope to motivate you to take ownership of their vascular health and begin on a journey of lifelong wellness by providing them with practical insights and tangible actions toward a heart-healthy lifestyle.

Conclusion

As I near the end of "Unveiling May-Thurner Syndrome: A Comprehensive Guide to Understanding and Managing Vascular Health," I reflect on the amount of material I have studied and the insights I have gained into the complex workings of the vascular system. From the perplexing nature of May-Thurner Syndrome to the broader context of vascular health and wellness, I have navigated difficult terrain using evidence-based research and clinical practice.

Throughout this book, our primary purpose has been to give you knowledge and insight so that you can make informed decisions about your vascular health and well-being. I have demystified a relatively unknown vascular condition and provided people with the tools they need to navigate the complexities of vascular medicine by throwing light on its cause, clinical symptoms, diagnostic approaches, and treatment options.

In addition to encouraging individual empowerment, I emphasized the need for vascular health advocacy and awareness-raising. May-Thurner Syndrome, like many other vascular illnesses, is frequently misdiagnosed or undetected, leading to delayed treatment and, in some cases, serious consequences. By raising awareness among healthcare professionals, patients, and the general public, I can ensure early discovery, prompt intervention, and better outcomes for those suffering from MTS and other vascular disorders.

As I leave these pages, I carry a renewed resolve to emphasize vascular health and wellness in our daily lives. I acknowledge the need to take proactive actions to maintain good vascular function and reduce the risk of cardiovascular disease, whether through regular exercise, a heart-healthy diet, stress management techniques, or proactive vascular screening.

Finally, I encourage you to put the information acquired from these pages into action, fighting for your vascular health and inspiring others to do the same.

As we part ways, I do so with a sense of optimism about the future of vascular medicine. May this book be a beacon of light in the field of vascular health, illuminating the route to better understanding, increased awareness, and, eventually, better results for people living with vascular disorders?